COMPLETE GUIDE TO UNDERSTANDING TONSILLECTOMY

Essential Insights, Benefits, Risks, Recovery Tips, And Post-Operative Care For A Successful Palatine Removal Surgery

KLEIN HOYLE

Disclaimer

The content in this book is based on the author's expertise and comprehension of the topic. The author has no affiliation or link with any corporation, business, or person. This book is meant to give general information and educational material only, and it should not be interpreted as professional medical advice. Always seek the advice of a skilled healthcare expert if you have any queries about medical issues or treatments. The author and publisher expressly disclaim any responsibility resulting directly or indirectly from the use or use of the information included in this book.

Table of Contents

ABOUT THIS BOOK

The "Complete Guide to Understanding Tonsillectomy" is an invaluable resource that gives in-depth insights into a treatment that affects the lives of many people. With rigorous attention to detail and a wealth of specialist information, this book is a source of clarity for patients, caregivers, and healthcare professionals alike.

Chapter 1 introduces readers to the essentials of tonsillectomy, including its definition, purpose, and historical background. This chapter provides a strong basis for understanding the importance of tonsillectomy in medical practice by diving into the anatomy of the tonsils and addressing typical causes for the treatment.

Chapter 2 discusses the indications for tonsillectomy, which include chronic tonsillitis, sleep apnea, and breathing issues. By outlining the numerous problems that may demand this surgical operation, this book enables readers to detect when tonsillectomy is appropriate and comprehend its possible advantages.

Preparation is critical, and Chapter 3 walks readers through the necessary measures for pre-surgery preparedness. From first consultations to psychological preparation, this chapter provides people with the information and resources they need to undertake the process confidently and clearly.

Chapter 4 gives a full explanation of the tonsillectomy operation, including the many kinds of surgeries accessible, the anesthetic process, and step-by-step surgical procedures. This chapter reduces anxiety and ensures that patients are fully informed throughout the surgical process by demystifying the procedure.

Post-operative care is critical, and Chapter 5 provides essential information on pain management, nutritional concerns, and recovery schedules. By explaining probable issues and when to seek medical assistance, this chapter prepares patients to navigate the post-surgical period with resilience and alertness.

Chapter 6 investigates the possible risks and problems related to tonsillectomy, providing practical advice on how to manage and reduce these issues. By discussing both frequent symptoms and unusual but important problems, this chapter encourages educated decision-making and proactive healthcare treatment.

Chapter 7 introduces readers to alternatives to tonsillectomy, enabling them to consider the advantages and disadvantages of various treatment choices. This chapter allows patients to make well-informed decisions that are tailored to their requirements and preferences by providing a detailed awareness of different techniques.

Chapter 8 focuses on pediatric concerns, delving into the particular problems and specialized treatment for young patients. From communication methods to recuperation recommendations, this chapter is important for caregivers navigating the tonsillectomy journey with children.

Chapter 9 dives into the complexity of adult tonsillectomy, including pain management, lifestyle changes, and long-term results. This chapter guarantees that people get individualized assistance and guidance throughout the rehabilitation process by recognizing their specific requirements as adults.

Finally, in Chapter 10, this book debunks myths and misunderstandings about tonsillectomy, providing evidence-based insights and credible sources for more information. By dispelling common fallacies and addressing worries and concerns, this chapter enables readers to approach tonsillectomy with clarity, confidence, and peace of mind.

CHAPTER 1

Introduction To Tonsillectomy

Definition And Function Of Tonsillectomy

Tonsillectomy is a surgical surgery that removes the tonsils, which are two oval-shaped tissues found in the back of the throat. This operation is often used to treat recurring throat infections, chronic tonsillitis, sleep apnea, and other associated issues. The main goal of a tonsillectomy is to reduce symptoms that severely impair a person's quality of life, such as difficulties breathing, swallowing problems, and repeated infections that do not respond to conventional treatment options.

The operation is often indicated when other therapies, such as antibiotics and medicines, have been unsuccessful.

Tonsillectomies may considerably decrease the incidence and severity of throat infections while improving general health and quality of life.

Historical Background

Tonsillectomy has a long and diverse history, with records extending back to antiquity. Roman doctors conducted the first known tonsillectomies circa 1000 BCE, utilizing basic instruments and procedures that were unpleasant and hazardous by modern standards. The process changed throughout the years as medical understanding and surgical skills advanced.

Tonsillectomy became a frequent practice in the nineteenth and early twentieth centuries, particularly in Western nations, as knowledge of infectious illnesses and their treatment improved. The development of anesthetic and antiseptic procedures in the late nineteenth century made surgery safer and more comfortable for patients.

Tonsillectomy is now a common surgical operation done under general anesthesia. Advances in surgical technology, such as the use of electrocautery and laser procedures, have helped to minimize risks and improve recovery periods.

Common Reasons For The Procedure

A tonsillectomy may be performed for a variety of reasons, the most prevalent of which are:

1. Recurrent Tonsillitis: Frequent inflammation of the tonsils, usually caused by bacteria or viral infections, resulting in painful throats, fever, and enlarged lymph nodes. When these infections persist numerous times per year and do not react well to medications, a tonsillectomy may be advised.

2. Obstructive sleep apnea occurs when enlarged tonsils impede the airway during sleep. This syndrome causes interrupted sleep, snoring, and other health

problems. Removing the tonsils may help clean the airway and enhance breathing while sleeping.

3. Chronic tonsillitis is a persistent inflammation of the tonsils that lasts many months, producing chronic pain and associated problems.

4. Tonsil stones (Tonsilloliths) are calcified material that collects in the tonsils' fissures, causing poor breath, painful throats, and trouble swallowing. In extreme circumstances, tonsil ectomy might bring relief.

5. A peritonsillar abscess is an accumulation of pus around the tonsil that may cause severe throat discomfort, fever, and trouble swallowing. If recurring, a tonsillectomy may be required to avoid future episodes.

Overview Of Tonsil Anatomy

Understanding the anatomy of the tonsils aids in grasping the causes and techniques for tonsillectomy. The tonsils are part of the body's immune system and are found in the throat. There are three types of tonsils:

1. **Palatine tonsils:** The most well-known and frequently removed during a tonsillectomy. When you open your mouth wide, you can see them on each side of the neck in the rear.

2. Pharyngeal Tonsils (Adenoids) is located on the roof of the nasopharynx, where the nose meets the throat. These are often not visible through the mouth and may be removed if they cause breathing difficulties or persistent infections.

3. **Lingual Tonsils:** Located at the base of the tongue. These are seldom removed, and primarily in situations when they cause sleep apnea or persistent infections.

The tonsils help to protect the body's immune system by capturing and filtering germs and viruses that enter via the mouth and nose. However, when the tonsils become a cause of recurring infections or substantial blockage, their removal is considered a desirable therapy option.

CHAPTER 2

Indications For Tonsillectomy

Chronic Tonsillitis

Chronic tonsillitis is a prolonged infection of the tonsils, which are two lymph nodes at the back of the throat. Unlike acute tonsillitis, which usually goes away after a few days of therapy, chronic tonsillitis lasts longer and frequently needs medical intervention. The illness may have a substantial impact on one's quality of life, causing chronic pain and recurring symptoms.

Patients with chronic tonsillitis have recurring sore throats, swollen and red tonsils, swallowing discomfort, and fevers. Inflammation may also result in white or yellow areas on the tonsils, suggesting pus production. Peritonsillar abscesses, or pus collections surrounding the tonsils, may form as a result of this prolonged illness.

These abscesses may cause significant discomfort, trouble swallowing, and, in certain circumstances, respiratory problems.

One of the main reasons for advocating a tonsillectomy in situations of chronic tonsillitis is to avoid recurring infections and their sequelae. The operation eliminates the cause of the infection, relieving symptoms and lowering the risk of future infections. Individuals who miss substantial amounts of school or work due to their symptoms may benefit from tonsillectomy since it eliminates the need for regular antibiotics and medical appointments.

Sleep Apnea And Breathing Problems

Sleep apnea is a dangerous sleep condition in which breathing stops and begins often during sleep. Tonsils, particularly when swollen, may restrict the airway and cause obstructive sleep apnea (OSA). Enlarged tonsils may obstruct airflow down the throat, resulting in snoring and spells of no breathing.

This illness is most frequent in youngsters, although it may also occur in adults.

Children with sleep apnea often display symptoms such as loud snoring, restless sleep, pauses in breathing, and daytime lethargy. Behavioral difficulties such as hyperactivity, trouble concentrating and poor academic performance are prevalent. If not addressed, sleep apnea in adults may cause serious health concerns such as high blood pressure, heart disease, and stroke.

A tonsillectomy may effectively cure sleep apnea caused by swollen tonsils. By eliminating the obstructive tissue, the airway is freed, allowing for regular breathing while sleeping. The technique may significantly enhance sleep quality, decrease snoring, and lower health risks. For youngsters, this may result in increased development, conduct, and academic achievement. Adults may benefit from improved cardiovascular health and general well-being.

Recurrent Strep Throat

Streptococcus pyogenes causes strep throat, which is characterized by discomfort and scratchiness. While strep throat is common and usually treated with medications, some people have recurrent infections, which are defined as several bouts within a single year. This may be physically and emotionally exhausting, requiring many physician appointments, lost school or work days, and several rounds of antibiotics.

Recurrent strep throat may also result in consequences like rheumatic fever, which causes inflammation in the heart, joints, and other tissues. Scarlet fever and renal inflammation are two more consequences of streptococcal infections. These dangers make controlling recurrent strep throat critical to overall health.

Tonsillectomy may be a very successful treatment for recurring strep throat. The frequency and severity of strep throat episodes may be greatly decreased by removing the tonsils, which contain the germs that cause the illness. This not only relieves the acute symptoms but also avoids the consequences that might arise from recurring infections. Patients who have a tonsillectomy for recurrent strep throat often report a significant improvement in their quality of life, including fewer sore throats, fewer antibiotics, and less time lost to sickness.

Tonsil Stones And Bad Breath

Tonsil stones, also known as tonsilloliths, are calcified deposits found in the tonsils' fissures. They consist of germs, dead cells, mucus, and other waste. While they are mostly innocuous, they may cause substantial pain and contribute to poor breath (halitosis). Tonsil stones may cause symptoms such as a sore throat, trouble swallowing, and earache.

Tonsil stones may cause bad breath, which can hurt social relationships and self-esteem. Coughing or physical removal may sometimes remove the stones, but they often reappear, resulting in a cycle of chronic suffering.

A tonsillectomy may provide a permanent treatment for those who have recurrent or big tonsil stones. The removal of the tonsils eliminates the environment that permits the stones to develop, preventing their recurrence. This may greatly enhance oral hygiene and general comfort. Patients often experience an immediate improvement in their breathing and a decrease in the pain associated with tonsil stones.

In conclusion, tonsillectomy is recommended for a variety of illnesses that have a major influence on a person's quality of life, such as chronic tonsillitis, sleep apnea, recurrent strep throat, and tonsil stones with poor breath. Each of these disorders may cause significant pain and health problems, making tonsillectomy a useful and often required procedure.

CHAPTER 3

Pre-Surgical Preparation

Initial Consultation And Medical History

The path to a tonsillectomy starts with an initial consultation with an otolaryngologist, sometimes known as an ENT (ear, nose, and throat) specialist. During this session, the doctor will go over your medical history in depth. This covers any past operations, chronic medical problems, current medicines, and known allergies. It is essential to give a thorough and accurate medical history so that the doctor can examine any possible hazards and establish if you are a good candidate for the surgery.

The doctor will also question about the symptoms that prompted you to contemplate a tonsillectomy. Common causes include recurring tonsillitis, sleep apnea, difficulties swallowing, and breathing issues. Be prepared to talk about the frequency, intensity, and duration of your symptoms. This information allows the clinician to better understand the effect of tonsillar disorders on your quality of life and make an educated choice about surgery.

Pre-Surgical Testing And Examinations

Before scheduling the tonsillectomy, many pre-surgical tests and exams are performed to assure the patient's safety and preparedness for surgery. These tests serve to discover any underlying disorders that may complicate the surgery.

1. **Physical Examination:** The ENT expert will do a comprehensive physical examination of the throat, ears, and nose. They will examine the tonsils' size and health, looking for infection or other abnormalities.

2. Blood tests are frequently conducted to look for anomalies in blood coagulation and to assess overall health. These tests may help uncover concerns such as

anemia or infection, which may need treatment before surgery.

3. Sleep Study: If sleep apnea is an issue, a sleep study may be advised. This entails spending the night in a sleep lab, where your breathing patterns, oxygen levels, and other vital indicators are recorded.

4. Imaging Tests: In certain circumstances, imaging tests such as X-rays or CT scans may be required to get a clear picture of the neck and surrounding tissues. This is particularly critical if there are anatomical problems that might jeopardize the procedure.

Diet And Medication Restrictions

In the weeks preceding the operation, you will be given precise dietary and pharmaceutical recommendations. These are critical for reducing the risk of problems during and after the treatment.

1. Drugs: Certain drugs, particularly those that impact blood coagulation, must be stopped before surgery.

This includes aspirin, nonsteroidal anti-inflammatory medications (NSAIDs), and some herbal supplements. Your doctor will give you a thorough list of drugs to avoid and may recommend alternatives if necessary.

2. Dietary Restrictions: You will be instructed not to eat or drink for a certain length of time before surgery, often beginning at midnight the night before the operation. This ensures that your stomach is empty, lowering the danger of aspiration (inhaling food or drinks into the lungs) during anesthesia.

3. Hydration: While solid food is limited, keeping hydrated is critical. Clear liquids such as water or electrolyte drinks may be permitted up to a few hours before surgery, but always adhere to the particular instructions advised by your healthcare team.

Psychological Preparation: Setting Expectations

Preparing mentally for a tonsillectomy is as crucial as physical preparation. Knowing what to anticipate might help alleviate anxiety and enhance overall results.

1. Understanding the operation: Learn more about the tonsillectomy operation. Understanding what will happen during surgery, the anesthetic procedure, and the projected recovery period may all assist in reducing concerns. Request that your doctor thoroughly describe the procedure's processes and give any written information or resources that are available.

2. Managing Anxiety: It is normal to feel worried before surgery. Deep breathing exercises, meditation, and talking to a counselor may all help you manage your anxiety before surgery. Relaxing activities such as reading, listening to music, or gentle exercise may all be useful.

3. Setting Realistic Expectations: Talk with your doctor about what you may reasonably anticipate in terms of recovery and results. Understanding the possible advantages, hazards, and usual recovery procedures might aid in setting reasonable expectations. Understanding that pain and recuperation are common components of the procedure will help you prepare psychologically and emotionally.

4. Support System: Arrange for assistance from family or friends throughout the healing phase. Having someone to help with everyday duties, emotional support, and transportation to and from the hospital may significantly improve your recovery experience.

By carefully following these pre-surgical preparation measures, you may ensure a smoother tonsillectomy experience with fewer risks and a better knowledge of the procedure, resulting in a more successful recovery.

CHAPTER 4

Tonsillectomy Procedure

Tonsillectomy Types: Traditional, Laser, And Coblation

Tonsillectomy, or surgical removal of the tonsils, may be done using a variety of procedures. Each treatment has advantages and disadvantages, and the process chosen is often determined by the surgeon's experience as well as the patient's requirements. There are three forms of tonsillectomy: traditional, laser, and collation.

Traditional Tonsillectomy

Traditional tonsillectomy involves the physician removing the tonsils with a knife or other surgical tools. This approach is typically regarded as the gold standard and has been utilized for many years. The tonsils are carefully separated from the surrounding tissues, and any bleeding is stopped using stitches, clamps, or electrocautery, which utilizes heat to close blood vessels.

Advantages:

• A widely performed and understood method.

• Effectively removes tonsil tissue.

Disadvantages:

• Can cause greater postoperative discomfort and longer recovery periods than other procedures.

• Increased risk of bleeding during and after surgery.

Laser Tonsillectomy

Laser tonsillectomy is the use of a laser to remove the tonsils. The laser slices through tissue while cauterizing blood arteries, which reduces bleeding.

Advantages:

• The laser's cauterizing impact led to less bleeding.

• Reduced surgical discomfort and speedier recovery.

Disadvantages:

• Needs specific equipment and training.

• Failure to do appropriately may result in burns or tissue damage.

Coblation Tonsillectomy

Coblation tonsillectomy creates a plasma field by combining radiofrequency radiation and a saline solution, which dissolves tonsil tissue at low temperatures. This approach lessens surgical discomfort while also minimizing tissue damage.

Advantages:

• Reduced surgical discomfort and quicker recovery than previous procedures.

• Reduced chance of tissue injury.

Disadvantages:

• Higher cost owing to specific equipment needed.

• Not as accessible as older ways.

Anesthesia: What To Expect

Tonsillectomy is usually done under general anesthesia, which means the patient is entirely sleeping and ignorant of the process. Understanding what to anticipate from anesthesia may help reduce anxiety and prepare for surgery.

Preoperative Preparation

Before anesthetic is administered, the patient is evaluated to determine that they are medically suitable for surgery. This involves a review of your medical history, allergies, and current medicines. The anesthesiologist will explain the anesthetic plan and answer any questions.

Induction of anesthesia

During the induction phase, an anesthetic is administered, often via an intravenous (IV) line. Patients may also be given a gas anesthetic using a mask. Within seconds or minutes, the patient will fall asleep.

Maintenance of anesthesia

Throughout the procedure, the anesthesiologist checks vital indicators such as heart rate, blood pressure, oxygen levels, and breathing. Anesthesia is maintained by administering IV drugs or inhaling gases to make the patient asleep and painless.

Emergence from Anesthesia

After the procedure, the anesthetic medications are discontinued, and the patient gradually awakens. This stage is carefully watched to ensure a smooth and safe recovery. Patients may first feel sluggish or confused.

Step-By-Step Surgical Procedure

Understanding the step-by-step process of a tonsillectomy may help to clarify the technique and offer insight into what occurs during surgery.

Step 1: Preoperative preparation

On the day of the operation, the patient reports to the hospital or surgical facility. Vital signs are examined, and an IV line is placed to give drugs and fluids. The patient is subsequently transported into the operating room.

Step 2: Induction of anesthesia

The patient is comfortably positioned on the surgical table. Anesthesia is injected, and the patient goes fast asleep. The anesthesiologist ensures that the patient is completely asleep and checks their status during the surgery.

Step 3: Tonsil exposure

Once the patient is anesthetized, the surgeon employs a mouth gag to hold the mouth open and expose the tonsils. A surgical lamp may be utilized to offer a good view of the tonsils.

Step 4: Remove Tonsils

The surgeon removes the tonsils using one of many methods, including conventional, laser, or coblation. A typical tonsillectomy involves dissecting the tonsils from the surrounding tissues. In a laser or coblation tonsillectomy, the tonsils are vaporized or removed.

Step 5: Hemostasis

After the tonsils are removed, the surgeon makes sure that all bleeding is under control. This might include cauterizing blood vessels or putting stitches in. Effective hemostasis is critical for preventing postoperative hemorrhage.

After the procedure is completed and the bleeding has been managed, the patient is gradually roused up from anesthesia. The patient is subsequently sent to a recovery room for intensive supervision.

Duration And Immediate Post-Operative Care

Duration of Surgery

The length of a tonsillectomy varies according to the procedure employed and the patient's circumstances. In most cases, the procedure lasts 30-60 minutes. However, the time spent in the operating room may be extended owing to anesthetic induction and recovery.

Immediate Post-Surgical Care

Following surgery, the patient is sent to a recovery room, where nurses check vital signs and general health.

The patient will stay in the recovery area until they are completely awake and stable. This first recuperation phase normally lasts between 1 and 2 hours.

Pain Management

Pain management is a key component of post-surgical treatment. To alleviate the patient's suffering, pain medicines will be administered. These may include oral pain medicines or, in certain situations, intravenous drugs. To promote a pleasant recovery, follow the pain management strategy as suggested.

Hydration and Nutrition

Staying hydrated is critical after a tonsillectomy. Initially, patients are recommended to consume clear fluids such as water, ice chips, and clear broth. They may gradually switch to soft, bland meals like applesauce, mashed potatoes, and yogurt. Avoiding hot, acidic, or hard meals may assist in reducing surgery site discomfort.

During the initial postoperative period, healthcare professionals keep an eye out for possible consequences such as bleeding, infection, and trouble breathing. Patients and caregivers are given guidance on what symptoms to look for and when to seek medical help.

Discharge Instructions:

Most tonsillectomies are conducted as outpatient procedures, which means patients may go home the same day. Before being discharged, patients are given thorough instructions on how to care for the surgical site, manage discomfort, and recognize indicators of problems. Follow-up sessions are planned to guarantee complete recovery.

Understanding the tonsillectomy technique, from the several kinds of operations offered to the anesthetic process, the step-by-step surgical process, and immediate post-surgery care, helps to demystify the experience and prepare patients and their caregivers for a more comfortable recovery.

CHAPTER 5

Post-Operative Care

Pain Management Techniques

After a tonsillectomy, pain management is critical for a good recovery. The pain is usually the most extreme in the first few days after surgery, then progressively subsides over two weeks. Here are some useful ways to manage pain:

Medications:

• Prescription Pain Relief: Your doctor may prescribe acetaminophen (Tylenol) or ibuprofen (Advil, Motrin). Serious pain may need the use of heavier drugs such as opioids.

• Non-prescription pain medicines such as acetaminophen or ibuprofen may be used, but it's important to follow dose directions from your healthcare professional.

• Timing and Consistency: Take pain medicine when recommended, rather than waiting until it becomes intolerable. Regular dosage helps to maintain a consistent degree of pain alleviation.

Cold therapy:

• Ice packs may relieve neck discomfort and swelling. Wrap the ice pack in a towel to prevent direct skin contact, then apply it at 20-minute intervals.

• Cold foods and drinks, such as popsicles, ice cream, and chilled beverages, may help soothe the throat.

Hydration:

• Stay Hydrated: Drinking lots of water may keep the throat moist and relieve pain. Choose cold or room-temperature beverages.

• Use a cool-mist humidifier in the bedroom to prevent throat dryness and discomfort during sleep.

• Provide enough rest to promote healing. Avoid talking and activities that may strain the throat.

Recommended Diet And Hydration

Proper diet and hydration are critical for healing after a tonsillectomy. The appropriate diet may help with healing, reducing pain, and preventing problems.

First few days:

• Start with clear drinks like water, apple juice, or broth. Gently introduce soft foods such as yogurt, pudding, mashed potatoes, and scrambled eggs.

• Ice cream, smoothies, and gelatin may provide relaxing effects. Avoid acidic, spicy, or rough-textured meals that might irritate the throat.

Hydration:

· Maintain proper hydration by drinking lots of water. Make an effort to consume 8–10 glasses of water every day. Popsicles and ice chips are also excellent choices.

• Avoid citrus fruits, fizzy drinks, and alcohol, which may cause throat inflammation.

Gradual Diet Progression:

• Introduce solid meals gradually as recovery proceeds. Begin with soft, easy-to-swallow meals and avoid anything crunchy or rough that might scrape the throat.

• Maintain a balanced diet with proteins, carbs, and fats to promote recovery. Consider making smoothies with fruits and veggies for extra nutrition.

Activity Restriction And Recovery Timeline

Post-operative care includes following activity limits and knowing the recovery period to enable good healing and prevent problems.

First week:

• Prioritize rest and minimize physical activity. Avoid intense activity and get plenty of sleep. To avoid bleeding and throat strain, limit your physical effort.

• Recovery requires at least one week away from school or work for most individuals. Follow your doctor's recommendations about when it is safe to return.

Second week:

• Gradual increase in activity: Return to usual activities as tolerated. Light walking is recommended to prevent blood clots but avoid heavy lifting, jogging, or strenuous activity.

• Pain Reduction: Pain should progressively subside over two weeks. Consult your doctor if the discomfort continues or worsens.

• Scab Formation and Healing: The surgical area will form a white or yellow scab as it heals. This is quite normal and should not be a concern.

• Typical recuperation time is two weeks, although some people may need more time. Follow all post-operative instructions and make follow-up visits to ensure optimal recovery.

Signs Of Complications And When To Get Help

Recognizing indicators of problems early is crucial for addressing any concerns quickly and ensuring a successful recovery. Contact your healthcare practitioner right away if you observe any of the following:

Bleeding:

• If there is severe or continuous bleeding from the neck, get medical treatment right once. Signs include bright red blood in the saliva and frequent swallowing.

• Vomiting blood or black, coffee-ground-like substance is a dangerous symptom that demands emergency medical attention.

Dehydration:
• Signs of dehydration include dry mouth, low urine flow, dark urine, and lethargy. Maintain enough fluid intake to avoid dehydration.

• A low fever is typical after surgery, but a prolonged high temperature (over 101.5°F or 38.6°C) might suggest an infection. If you get a high temperature, please contact your doctor.

Severe pain

• Consult your healthcare practitioner if pain persists or worsens despite medication.

Difficulty breathing:

• Breathing problems or edema should be treated as an emergency. Seek emergency medical care.

Persistent vomiting:

• Persistent vomiting might cause dehydration and need medical attention.

Understanding these indicators and following post-operative care recommendations can help you recover safely and smoothly after a tonsillectomy. Always follow your healthcare provider's advice and do not be afraid to seek assistance if any problems emerge throughout the healing process.

CHAPTER 6

Potential Risks And Complications

Common Post-Surgery Symptoms

Pain and discomfort

Pain is one of the most prevalent post-tonsillectomy complaints for people. This discomfort is usually felt in the throat, but it may sometimes go to the ears, a condition called referred pain. The pain may worsen when swallowing, making it difficult to eat or drink. Over-the-counter pain medicines such as acetaminophen are often advised, but stronger drugs may be required for severe pain. To successfully treat pain, these drugs must be taken exactly as prescribed.

Swelling and inflammation

Swelling of the throat and uvula is another typical postoperative symptom. This swelling may worsen the discomfort and make swallowing harder.

Ice packs placed externally to the neck might help minimize swelling. In rare circumstances, a doctor may prescribe steroids to reduce inflammation and help in the healing process.

Scabs and Throat Appearance

As the surgical areas in the throat heal, white or yellowish scabs appear where the tonsils are removed. This is a natural aspect of the healing process. However, these scabs may sometimes result in poor breath and an unpleasant taste in the mouth. It is critical to avoid picking at these scabs or eating tough foods that may dislodge them early since this might result in bleeding.

Changes in Voice

Following a tonsillectomy, temporary voice alterations are frequent. This might include a nasal voice or a minor shift in tone. These alterations often fade when the throat recovers, which usually takes a few weeks.

Due to the discomfort and swelling, many patients find it difficult to eat or drink for many days after surgery. Staying hydrated is crucial, so drinking water, ice chips, and clear broths may assist. Soft foods, such as yogurt, mashed potatoes, and applesauce, may be offered gradually as tolerance develops.

Rare Yet Serious Complications

Hemorrhage

One of the most dangerous risks of a tonsillectomy is post-operative bleeding, which may occur within 24 hours or up to 10 days following surgery. This sort of bleeding often occurs at the surgical site where the scabs have fallen off early. Spitting up bright red blood or having a lot of blood in your vomit are both signs of hemorrhage. If this happens, you must seek emergency medical assistance since severe blood loss may be fatal.

Infection

While infections are uncommon, they may develop and disrupt the healing process. Symptoms of an infection include fever, increasing throat discomfort, and swelling that seems to worsen rather than improve. Contact your physician if you think you may have an infection. They may prescribe medications to treat the illness and avoid consequences.

Anesthesia Reactions

Although uncommon, reactions to anesthesia may develop during or after surgery. These responses may include nausea, vomiting, or, in very rare situations, more serious consequences such as breathing trouble. To reduce risk, discuss any past anesthetic reactions with your surgeon before the treatment.

Breathing difficulties

In rare cases, swelling in the throat after surgery might create breathing problems. This is especially problematic in young children since their airways are smaller. If you or your kid has difficulties breathing, get emergency medical attention immediately.

Managing Bleeding And Infection Risks

Pre-Surgical Preparation

Proper preparation before surgery may help reduce the risk of bleeding and infection. This includes any pre-operative advice from your healthcare physician, such as discontinuing certain drugs that raise bleeding risk. Additionally, regular dental hygiene may minimize the bacterial load in the mouth, minimizing the risk of illness.

Post-Surgical Care

Post-operative care is crucial for minimizing bleeding and infection concerns. Make sure you follow all post-surgery instructions provided by your healthcare professional.

This often entails taking prescribed medicines, following dietary advice, and avoiding intense activities that may disturb the surgery sites.

Monitoring and Follow-up

Regular monitoring of your health after surgery is critical. Pay close attention to any changes in your symptoms, particularly evidence of bleeding or infection. Schedule and attend any follow-up visits with your healthcare practitioner to ensure appropriate healing and timely resolution of any issues.

Emergency measures

Knowing when to seek emergency treatment is critical. If you are experiencing severe pain, major bleeding, a high temperature, or trouble breathing, please call emergency services right once. Early intervention may avert significant problems and improve results.

Long-Term Health Considerations

Immune System Impact

The tonsils are part of the body's immune system, which helps it fight illnesses. While their removal has no major influence on overall immune function, it may increase vulnerability to throat infections temporarily. uptime, the body adjusts, and other tissues take up the immunological activities that the tonsils used to do.

Speech & Swallowing

Long-term impacts on speech and swallowing are often negligible. Most patients recover normal function after a few weeks or months of surgery. However, in rare situations, some people may endure lasting alterations in voice or swallowing, which may be addressed with speech therapy if necessary.

Sleep and Breathing

Those who have undergone a tonsillectomy to treat obstructive sleep apnea or chronic tonsillitis may see considerable improvements in their sleep quality and breathing. Many patients report fewer sleep disturbances and better overall health after recovery.

Recurring Throat Issues

A tonsillectomy may lessen the incidence of throat infections, but it does not ensure that they will never return. Maintaining proper dental hygiene and general health habits is critical to avoiding future problems.

Lifestyle Adjustments

Adapting to life after a tonsillectomy requires certain short-term and maybe long-term lifestyle changes. Initially, this entails maintaining a soft diet while gradually reintroducing conventional meals. Long-term, it entails being mindful of throat health and obtaining immediate medical attention for any new difficulties that occur.

Patients might be more confident and prepared for their tonsillectomy if they understand the possible dangers and problems, as well as how to manage them.

CHAPTER 7

Alternatives To Tonsillectomy

Nonsurgical Treatments

When contemplating tonsillectomy, it is critical to look into non-surgical options that may ease symptoms without the need for surgery. Medication is a frequent nonsurgical treatment option. Antibiotics are often administered to treat bacterial infections that cause tonsillitis. These drugs may help eliminate the infection and decrease inflammation, relieving symptoms including a sore throat and trouble swallowing.

Corticosteroids are a non-surgical therapy option. These drugs may help decrease inflammation and swelling in the tonsils, alleviating symptoms including discomfort and trouble breathing.

Corticosteroids may be given orally or as injections, depending on the severity of the symptoms.

In addition to medicine, non-surgical therapies for a sore throat include gargling with salt water and using throat lozenges. These easy solutions may help alleviate throat pain and irritation, making it easier to swallow and talk.

Watchful Waiting Approach

Some people, particularly youngsters, may benefit from a cautious waiting strategy rather than rapid surgery. This method entails monitoring the disease over time to observe whether the symptoms improve on their own or worsen. During this time of observation, healthcare experts may advise on supportive measures such as rest, water, and pain treatment to assist relieve symptoms.

The cautious waiting method is especially popular in children with recurring tonsillitis. Because tonsillitis usually improves as children become older and their immune systems develop surgery may be avoided if the symptoms are not severe or frequent. However, if symptoms continue or increase over time, surgery may be reconsidered.

Advantages And Disadvantages Of Alternatives

Nonsurgical therapy and the careful waiting strategy have significant advantages over tonsillectomy. These methods are often less intrusive and have less hazards than surgery. Furthermore, they may be more appropriate for those who choose not to have surgery or who have underlying health issues that make surgery unsafe.

However, non-surgical therapies and the careful waiting strategy both have downsides. For example, medicines may only give temporary relief from symptoms and may not treat the underlying cause of tonsillitis. Similarly, the careful waiting strategy requires continual observation and may increase pain if symptoms do not improve.

Determining The Best Course Of Action

Choosing the optimal tonsillectomy treatment takes careful evaluation of the patient's medical history, symptoms, and preferences. Healthcare experts will evaluate the severity and frequency of tonsillitis bouts, as well as any complications or underlying medical issues that may influence treatment choices.

Finally, the choice to seek surgery or non-surgical options should be made collectively by the person, their family, and their healthcare professional. It is critical to consider the possible advantages and hazards of each strategy and choose the one that provides the highest possibility of symptom alleviation and a better quality of life.

CHAPTER 8

Pediatric Considerations

Tonsillectomy Differences In Pediatrics And Adults

Tonsillectomy, or surgical removal of the tonsils, is a frequent surgery in both pediatric and adult populations. However, there are numerous major distinctions between conducting tonsillectomies on children and adults.

First, the size of the tonsils varies greatly between children and adults. Children's tonsils are often bigger in proportion to their throat size than adults. This might complicate the surgical operation in pediatric patients because the surgeon must maneuver around bigger tonsils in a limited area.

Furthermore, the grounds for tonsillectomies might vary between children and adults. Tonsillectomies are often done in children to treat the symptoms of recurrent throat infections or obstructive sleep apnea caused by swollen tonsils. Adults, on the other hand, may have a tonsillectomy to treat persistent tonsillitis or complications such as abscesses.

Another crucial factor is the recuperation procedure. Children heal quicker than adults after tonsillectomy. This is due in part to young people's resilience and the fact that youngsters recover faster than adults. However, parents should continue to monitor their child's recovery and adhere to the surgeon's post-operative care guidelines.

Special Care For Children Before And After Surgery

Preparing a kid for a tonsillectomy requires specific measures to guarantee their comfort and safety before, during, and after the surgery.

Before surgery, parents should talk with their kids about what to anticipate. This involves describing the cause for the operation in age-appropriate language and responding to any worries or anxieties the kid may have. In addition, the healthcare team will offer advice on fasting before surgery and any drugs that should be avoided.

Pediatric patients are usually given general anesthetic during surgery to keep them motionless and comfortable. The surgeon will gently remove the tonsils with specialist devices, taking care to avoid bleeding and harm to the surrounding tissues.

Children may be uncomfortable and have difficulties swallowing for many days after surgery. It is critical for parents to regularly check their children's discomfort levels and encourage them to drink lots of water. Soft, chilled foods like ice cream or yogurt may also help soothe the throat and give nourishment throughout the healing process.

Communicating With Children About The Procedure

Talking to children about tonsillectomy may be difficult, but open and honest communication is vital for calming worries and making them feel educated and supported.

When discussing the operation with a youngster, be sure to use age-appropriate language and explanations. Avoid using medical jargon and instead, describe the operation in basic words that people can comprehend. Use visual aids, such as images or diagrams, to assist explain the procedure and answer any questions they may have.

Assure the kid that the operation is being conducted to make them feel better and relieve any pain they may be suffering as a result of swollen tonsils. Emphasize that the healthcare staff will care for them before, during, and after the surgery, and that they will be continuously monitored to ensure a smooth recovery.

Encourage the youngster to communicate their thoughts and worries about the operation, and validate their emotions by recognizing their anxieties and reminding them that being frightened is acceptable. Provide lots of support and encouragement during the process, and remind them that they are not alone - their parents, caretakers, and healthcare professionals are there to assist them every step of the way.

Recovery Tips For Young Patients

Tonsillectomy recovery may be difficult for children, but there are various measures parents can employ to help their kids feel better and heal faster.

First and foremost, attentively follow the surgeon's post-operative care recommendations. This may involve giving pain medicine as directed, keeping an eye out for indications of bleeding or infection, and recommending lots of rest.

Cold and soft foods like popsicles, ice cream, yogurt, or smoothies might help relieve throat pain and discomfort. Avoid offering your kid acidic or spicy meals that might irritate their throats, and urge them to remain hydrated by drinking lots of water.

Maintain your child's comfort by establishing a relaxing atmosphere at home. Use a cool-mist humidifier to bring moisture to the air and relieve throat dryness, and offer lots of soft pillows and blankets so they can sleep comfortably.

Encourage moderate hobbies like reading, drawing, or watching movies to keep your youngster occupied while they heal. Avoid intense activity or rough play that might cause injury or bleeding.

Follow your child's recovery carefully and call your healthcare practitioner if you have any concerns or observe any indications of problems, such as severe bleeding, fever, or trouble breathing.

CHAPTER 9

Adult Tonsillectomy Insights

Adult Patients Have Unique Challenges

Adult tonsillectomy presents significant complications as compared to the treatment in minors. One notable distinction is that adults have a higher risk of problems owing to variables such as bigger tonsils, more developed blood arteries, and possibly underlying health concerns. The surgical approach may need to be modified to account for these variations and reduce hazards.

Furthermore, adults may have a greater tolerance for pain and discomfort, making post-operative pain management critical. Adults may also take longer to recover owing to slower healing and the possibility of complications such as bleeding or infection. Thus, close monitoring and suitable treatments are required to guarantee a smooth healing phase.

Furthermore, adult patients may have commitments such as employment or caring for family members, which might limit their capacity to relax and recover after surgery. To address these issues, a thorough strategy must be taken that takes into account the unique requirements and circumstances of each adult patient having a tonsillectomy.

Pain Management And Recovery Differences

Pain management is an important part of adult tonsillectomy since there is a risk of considerable pain after surgery. Adults often feel more extreme pain and discomfort than children, which may hurt their quality of life throughout the recovery period.

To successfully treat pain, a mix of drugs and non-pharmacological measures might be used. Prescription pain medicines, over-the-counter analgesics, and treatments such as cold therapy or throat lozenges may also be used to ease discomfort.

Furthermore, adults may need extra assistance throughout recuperation to ensure proper rest and water. To avoid dehydration and improve recovery, dietary changes such as eating softer meals and drinking more fluids may be necessary.

Understanding the variations in pain perception and recovery between adults and children allows healthcare practitioners to adjust their approach to the individual requirements of adult tonsillectomy patients.

Impact On Adult Lifestyle And Work

The choice to get a tonsillectomy as an adult might have a considerable influence on your lifestyle and professional duties. Unlike children, who may have greater scheduling flexibility, adults often have professional and personal commitments that must be addressed before surgery.

Tonsillectomy recovery may include taking time off work or adjusting tasks to account for decreased energy and probable pain. Adults must address these factors with their healthcare professional and employer to make suitable plans and promote a seamless return to regular activities.

Furthermore, lifestyle changes may be required throughout the recovery time, such as avoiding vigorous activities or social gatherings that might hamper healing. Open communication with family and friends may be very helpful at this time.

Long-Term Results And Follow-Up Care

Understanding the long-term results and possible problems of adult tonsillectomy is critical for making educated decisions and providing follow-up treatment. While the operation may alleviate chronic tonsillitis or other underlying diseases, there are risks connected with surgery that may need continued monitoring and care.

Scarring, changes in voice quality, or tonsil tissue regrowth are all possible long-term consequences that need frequent follow-up meetings with healthcare experts. Monitoring for symptoms of infection or other post-operative problems is also critical to ensuring prompt management and best results.

Furthermore, resolving any residual problems or concerns after surgery is critical to adult patients' general well-being. This might include obtaining assistance from an otolaryngologist or other healthcare specialists to handle any concerns that occur throughout the healing process.

Patients may make educated choices and get the support they need for a successful recovery by knowing the specific obstacles, pain management options, lifestyle concerns, and long-term results related to adult tonsillectomy.

CHAPTER 10
Myths And Misconceptions

Dispelling Common Myths About Tonsillectomy

Tonsillectomy is often associated with myths and misunderstandings, which may create undue concern and uncertainty for patients and families. A prevalent misconception is that tonsillectomy is a risky treatment with serious consequences. Tonsillectomy is a generally safe procedure when done by a trained and experienced surgeon in a recognized medical institution. Like any operation, there are dangers, but the benefits often exceed the risks, particularly for those who suffer from recurrent tonsillitis or other issues caused by swollen or inflamed tonsils.

Another fallacy is that tonsillectomies are exclusively done on children. While tonsillectomy is most typically done on children, adults may also benefit from the treatment, particularly if they have chronic tonsillitis or obstructive sleep apnea. Adults may be at a greater risk of chronic tonsillitis issues because their tonsils are bigger and their airways are smaller.

Some people assume that tonsillectomy is a painful treatment that requires a lengthy and tough recovery. While tonsillectomy may cause some pain, advances in surgical methods and post-operative care have made the healing period considerably easier for patients. Pain management techniques, such as medicines and tongue lozenges, may help ease pain, and most patients can return to regular activities within a week or two after surgery.

Evidence-Based Facts

When contemplating tonsillectomy, it is critical to base your decision on evidence-based information. Numerous studies have shown that tonsillectomy improves the quality of life for those with chronic tonsillitis or obstructive sleep apnea. For example, tonsillectomy has been proven in studies to greatly decrease the frequency and severity of sore throats and upper respiratory infections in children and adults with recurrent tonsillitis.

Similarly, tonsillectomy has been demonstrated to be a successful therapy for obstructive sleep apnea in both children and adults. Tonsillectomy, which removes the swollen tonsils that impede the airway during sleep, may improve breathing and lower the risk of sleep apnea symptoms such as daytime weariness and cardiovascular difficulties.

Addressing Fears And Concerns

It is normal to have doubts and concerns regarding any surgical surgery, including tonsillectomy. However, it is critical to address these anxieties and concerns with appropriate information and guidance from healthcare experts.

Patients should feel comfortable asking questions and expressing their concerns to their surgeons and medical staff.

One prevalent concern is the possibility of complications during or after a tonsillectomy. While problems are conceivable, they are uncommon, particularly when the treatment is done by a qualified surgeon in a controlled setting. Common consequences include bleeding, infection, and anesthesia-related responses, although these risks may be reduced with careful pre-operative and post-operative care.

Another worry is how tonsillectomy affects everyday living, such as eating, speech, and activities. While there may be some temporary changes, such as difficulty swallowing or speaking properly right after surgery, most patients may return to regular activities within a week or two. To ensure a smooth recovery, follow the surgeon's post-operative instructions, which may include food restrictions and activity limits.

Reliable Resources For Further Information

There are various credible sites accessible for anyone interested in learning more about tonsillectomy. Trusted medical websites, such as those run by recognized hospitals or academic organizations, may give thorough information regarding the surgery, recuperation time, and possible dangers and advantages.

Patients may also seek tailored information and suggestions from their primary care physician or an otolaryngologist. These healthcare specialists may analyze an individual's risk factors and medical history to decide if tonsillectomy is the best option, as well as give support during the decision-making and healing process.

Overall, by refuting common beliefs, relying on evidence-based facts, addressing worries and concerns, and exploring credible resources for further information, people may make educated choices regarding tonsillectomy and be confident in their treatment.

Conclusion

Understanding tonsillectomy is critical for both patients and caretakers. This thorough guide has covered all elements of tonsillectomy, from the indications to the surgical method, post-operative care, and possible consequences. Individuals who are equipped with this information may approach the operation with confidence and manage the recovery process more successfully.

First and foremost, it is critical to understand the indications for tonsillectomy. Understanding why surgery is necessary, whether for recurrent tonsillitis, obstructive sleep apnea, or other major consequences, gives patients clarity and peace of mind. Furthermore, understanding the alternatives to tonsillectomy enables patients to make educated choices regarding their treatment options in cooperation with their doctors.

Understanding the surgical technique is another crucial factor. From pre-operative preparations to the anesthetic process and surgical methods used, knowing what to anticipate throughout the procedure reduces anxiety and fosters a feeling of readiness. Furthermore, being aware of the possible dangers and consequences connected with tonsillectomy emphasizes the necessity of choosing a knowledgeable surgeon and following post-operative instructions carefully.

Post-operative care is critical for a successful recovery. Patients and caregivers must be cautious during the first few days after surgery, from managing pain and discomfort to keeping an eye out for bleeding or infection. Understanding the food restrictions, activity constraints, and medication regimen given by healthcare practitioners promotes optimum recovery and lowers the risk of problems.

Furthermore, understanding the projected period for recovery is critical for establishing reasonable expectations. While some people recuperate quickly in a week or two, others may take many weeks to completely recover. Individuals may better navigate the postoperative phase if they understand the variety in healing rates and are patient with the procedure.

A thorough knowledge of tonsillectomy enables patients and caregivers to make educated choices, actively engage in their healthcare journey, and achieve optimal results. Individuals who are knowledgeable about the reasons, surgical method, post-operative care, and possible risks may approach tonsillectomy with confidence and ease the healing process. Maintaining open communication with healthcare practitioners, as well as seeking support from family and friends, may all contribute to a positive overall experience and result.

THE END